NUTRIBULLET Recipe Book

Mouth-watering Smoothie Recipes for Weight Loss, Detox, De stress, controlling Diabetes and Looking and Feeling Great.

By Caroline G.Hawley

Table of contents

Disclaimer

The recipes provided in this report are for informational purposes only and are not intended to provide dietary advice. A medical practitioner should be consulted before making any changes in diet. Additionally, recipe cooking times may require adjustment depending on age and quality of appliances. Readers are strongly urged to take all precautions to ensure ingredients are fully cooked in order to avoid the dangers of food borne viruses. The recipes and suggestions provided in this book are solely the opinion of the author. The author and publisher do not take any responsibility for any consequences that may result due to following the instructions provided in this book.

INTRODUCTION

The NUTRiBULLET is no simple blending appliance, it ensures that you get every single drop of goodness from the fruits and vegetables you morph into smoothies. The handy-dandy little machine has got horse power enough to make your lawn mower jealous and that's why it has the unique ability to extract nutrients from every single part of your fruits and vegetables including the skin, pulp and seeds.

The 1700-watt version can convert your ingredients into a smoothie in a few seconds flat, leaving just a simple, smooth, satisfying drink. If you're ready to upgrade life as you know it, then it's time to get friendly with your NUTRiBULLET.

You make many important decisions daily, but one of them is critical in determining the overall quality of your day and your life on the whole. Whether it's breakfast, lunch, dinner or snacks, the quality of the food you decide to eat has a direct impact on your performance in all areas of your life.

And that is why it is so important that you're consuming foods that are going to help you instead of hurt you. Foods that are going to help are foods like fruits and vegetables and nuts because they're chock full of nutrients the body needs. The best way to eat most of your fruits and veggies is whole and raw and also preferably organic.

And one of the best ways to consume the amount of fruits and veggies you need daily is in the form of a clean smoothie. Drinking whole food smoothies means you're able to get a lot more fruits and veggies into your body then you would if you were to consume each one individually.

Sometimes people forget that the reason we consume food is because it contains important nutrients that the body needs in order to function. The minute we start viewing food for its pleasure value only instead of its function, it is then that health problems begin and the aging process goes into overdrive.

Clean, whole, natural foods have everything you need to fuel your body for optimal living. The NUTRiBULLET Recipe Book has been specifically designed to help ensure that you're getting a big, healthy dose of those very natural foods.

As you increase your consumption of the smoothies in this book you'll notice a happier, more energetic you. Your skin will be brighter, you'll feel lighter and any mental muddling will be a thing of the past.

Clean smoothies can indeed detoxify your body and give you a new lease on life.

Chapter 1: How to make smoothies with your NUTRiBULLET

Make it organic

The most important decision you're going to make when making your perfect smoothie is in regards to the type of ingredients you're going to use. In the coming chapters you're going to find recipes to suit just about any requirement you have from beauty goals to weight loss goals, however the quality of ingredient that you use will determine how well the smoothie accomplishes what it's been designed to do for you.

You see, not all fruits and vegetables are made equal despite what they make look like on the outside. Your standard grocery store fruits and veggies can contain all sorts of herbicides, fungicides and insecticide which are essentially composed of harmful chemicals.

Up until the Industrial Revolution you could feel confident that when you purchased fruits and veggies you were getting clean, wholesome goods grown with the help of water and sunshine. However, with the world shrinking and mass production becoming the norm rather than the exception, all sorts of chemical agents were introduced to ensue crops were not ruined by insects and that in fact they grew faster and stronger.

Although the chemicals weren't instantly embraced by all producers, they slowly did become the norm due to competition. A farmer that didn't use the chemicals had smaller crops, crops that occasionally failed and imperfect produce as is normal in the case of nature.

However, these farmers were competing with other producers that ensured their crops were better protected from nuisance insects and plants, thereby ensuring larger crops with little visible imperfections.

These days, standard fruits and vegetables offered in your local grocery store are going to contain some type of chemical. You can avoid these chemical-laden fruits and vegetables by buying organic. Yes, organic goods will be more expensive than regular fruits and veggies and for good reason. Fruits and veggies labelled organic must follow strict rules during the planting and growing process in order to ensure the products are free of harmful substances.

Although chemicals are found in most standard grocery store fruits and vegetables, fruits tend to have a higher amount of chemicals than vegetables for the most part. Fruits are more sensitive to extreme weather conditions, easily damaged and are more often the target of insects and foraging animals. Since fruits are so sensitive and the chance of having a bad crop so high, a lot more chemicals are used on them to help them along.

Although vegetables are heartier than fruit and can withstand more rough treatment than fruits, the name of the farming game is perfection. Therefore, most veggies you're going to find on your grocery shelves will contain harmful chemical strains. In light of the aforementioned facts, it is always a good idea to buy organic and if you can buy locally organic it's even better.

Of course, folks have budget constraints and buying organic is more expensive, but it's better to buy less and ensure you're putting high quality food in your body. Overall, if you do find yourself a little strained on budget, check out the list below of the most dangerous fruits and veggies, and buy those in the organic section. Items that do not appear on the list can be purchased in the non-organic section when the budget calls for it.

Fruit & Vegetable Danger List

You should be particularly wary of purchasing the following fruits and vegetables from the standard produce section. The items on this list are often found to contain the highest strain of pesticides according to a variety of agencies including the US Environmental Watchdog Agency (EWA).

Apple

Strawberry

Peach

Grape

Nectarine

Bell Peppers

Celery

Cherry tomatoes

Snap Peas

Spinach

How Organic Helps with Detox

Most people just starting out with the NUTRiBULLET often use it as an opportunity to kick-start a new healthy lifestyle and that new lifestyle often begins with a detox. If you're planning on a smoothie detox than it is of particular importance that you use organic ingredients rather than those from the standard section of your grocery store.

Going on a total smoothie detox helps to overhaul your bodily systems by getting rid of the toxin build-up. The cleanse then let's you start your new healthy lifestyle with a clean slate.

However, if you're detoxing with smoothies that are made up of fruits and veggies that contain toxins, you're not going to get the full benefit of the detox. You will get rid of toxins, but you'll also be adding toxins via toxic fruits and veggies. In the case of a detox, we recommend you stick with organic in order to obtain a total cleanse.

NUTRiBULLET cheat sheet

- Before you do anything else, thoroughly scrub and wash your vegetables and fruit as needed to get rid of any residue.

- Next, seed and core as needed and give your fruits and/or veggies a rough chop, you don't have to be too precise since the NUTRiBULLET is powerful enough to extract and pulverize even the largest of chunks.

  Place your veggies into the NUTRiBULLET first and top those with your fruits. Next add the dry ingredients you're using like protein powder, nuts, seeds and spices. Lastly, add your liquids like water or milk and ice if you want a chilled smoothie.

- Your NUTRiBULLET comes with two blades, one is for extracting and the other one is for turning dry ingredients like nuts into fine granules. You're going to use the extract blade, which is sharp on both sides, screw this on top of your NUTRiBULLET lid.

- Plug your NUTRiBULLET base into an electric socket and place your cup onto the base and whip up your smoothie.

- Remove the cup from the base and shake it, if it's too thick add liquid and give it another turn on the base.

- You can drink your smoothie right out of the NUTRiBULLET cup if you would like or pour it into another cup and place the NUTRiBULLET into your dishwasher for easy clean-up.

- Clean the base of the NUTRiBULLET with a cloth that is slightly damp and wash the blade with soap and water.

- And that's how you create the perfectly simple and perfectly delicious smoothie with your NUTRiBULLET.

Got Nutrients?

Let's be honest, most of us don't come anywhere close to eating the amounts of fruits and veggies we should on a daily basis. Sometimes it can simply feel like you just don't have time to fit 6-8 servings of fruits and veggies into your day, not when there's all that other stuff to eat.

Smoothies are a brilliant way to get all those fruits and veggies you should be eating into a glass or two. You can easily get 4 servings of nutrient-rich fruits and veggies into a NUTRiBULLET glass if not more. Drinking your daily dose of nutrients is a lot quicker and easier than carting around a bushel of apples to eat throughout your day. Incorporating smoothies into your diet makes eating right a little bit easier.

Get Gorgeous

Fruits and vegetables contain a ton of antioxidants and you need those antioxidants to chase the free radicals right out of your body. Free radicals are responsible for putting strain on your cells and aging you.

Antioxidants go into your body and fight the radicals off so your cells can live in peace. You will notice a significant improvement in your skin after drinking smoothies for a week, there will be a certain glow that wasn't there before.

Healthy noshing to-go

Sometimes it seems near impossible to eat healthy when you're on the go. Often times your quick food choices are limited to fast food, gas station snacks or junk food like chips, cookies and candy.

However, once your incorporate smoothies into your diet you won't have that problem any longer. You can easily whip up a double batch of your smoothie, drink one at home and take the second one t go.

A smoothie can be a complete meal replacement thanks to all the nutrients it can contain.

Lose weight

If you go on a smoothie cleans, you're going to see the pounds just sliding off without much effort from you. Of course, it is possible to make unhealthy smoothies by using ingredients like ice cream, sugars and processed flavorings. But if you're going to make the real smoothies we've provided in this book, you're going to lose weight.

Even if you incorporate the smoothies into your diet instead of a cleanse, you'll still see weight loss because our smoothies are made up of the cleanest ingredients. Because the smoothies provided in this book are nutrient-dense you'll stay full longer and have no urge to snack too.

Detoxify

Going on a 3-day, 5-day or 7-day smoothie cleanse will do all sorts of amazing things for your body. You will actually feel the difference between your pre-detox and post-detox body. Replacing your meals with good, clean smoothies will give your body a chance to clean house since you won't be adding new toxins into your system.

All of the liquid you will be drink combined with the anti-oxidant goodness will flush your system of all the junk and leave you feeling clean and clear and only then will you realize how sluggish you were feeling before.

High Energy

The smoothie recipes provided in this book are made up of ingredients that are alive for the most part. Alive ingredients are those that aren't processed, aren't cooked, essentially they're in their natural state. Because you're ingesting food that is alive, you'll notice that the energy that you get from it is of a richer kind. A smoothie or two a day will increase your energy levels and make you actually feel more alive.

Chapter 3: Weight Loss Smoothies

Smoothies make it easy for you to shed pounds while keeping satiated. That's right, it is possible to feel full while substituting one of your daily meals with a smoothie. And not only are you satiated, but you're likely getting more nutrients than if you were to sit down to a meal. How is that possible?

The following batch of smoothies have been specifically designed to help you slash weight while ensuring you're getting all of the nutrients that you need. Since your smoothies are composed of whole foods and since the NUTRiBULLET is able to utilize all components of your whole foods from skin to seed, you're going to do your body good. Now, there are several ways to lose weight with smoothies, you can go low-cal or you can go high fat low-carb.

In this section we'll provide you with low-cal, high-fiber smoothies that will allow you to do a total cleanse and in turn help you drop that weight you've been holding.

The Super Green Smoothie

Serves: 2

Prep Time: 5 minutes

Ingredients

4 cups raw spinach

½ English cucumber

¼ cup mint leaves

2 lemons, juiced

1 apple, peeled, cored

½ cup ice.

Directions

- ○ Steam spinach.
- ○ Combine spinach with remaining ingredients in NUTRiBULLET, mix until smooth.

Nutrition (g)

Calories 94

Fat 1

Sodium 56 (mg)

Carbs 24

Fiber 6

Sugars 12

Protein 4

The Tropics Smoothie

Serves: 2

Prep Time: 5 minutes

Ingredients

½ cup pineapple

1 banana

¾ cup 1 percent milk

½ cup ice

¼ tsp vanilla extract

Directions

- o Place ingredients in NUTRiBULLET and mix until smooth.

Nutrition (g)

Calories 116

Fat 1

Sodium 52 (mg)

Carbs 24

Fiber 2

Sugars 16

Protein 4

Celery Twist

Serves: 2

Prep Time: 5 minutes

Ingredients

2 stalks celery

2 carrots

¾ cup tomato juice

½ tsp Tabasco sauce

½ tsp salt

½ cup ice

Directions

- o Place ingredients in NUTRiBULLET and mix until smooth.

Nutrition (g)

Calories 43

Fat 0

Sodium 884 (mg)

Carbs 10

Fiber 2

Sugars 7

Protein 1

Refreshing Mint Smoothie

Serves: 2

Prep Time: 5 minutes

Ingredients

½ cup mint leaves

1 tsp wheatgrass

1 green apple, peeled, cored

2 lemons, juiced

½ cup coconut water

½ cup ice

Directions

- o Place ingredients in NUTRiBULLET and mix until smooth.

Nutrition (g)

Calories 85

Fat 0

Sodium 49 (mg)

Carbs 20

Fiber 5

Sugars 14

Protein 2

Blueberry Yogurt Smoothie

Serves: 2

Prep Time: 5 minutes

Ingredients

1 cup frozen blueberries

½ cup oatmeal, cooked

½ cup low-fat yogurt

Directions

- o Place ingredients in NUTRiBULLET and mix until smooth.

Nutrition (g)

Calories 85

Fat 0

Sodium 49 (mg)

Carbs 20

Fiber 5

Sugars 14

Protein 2

The Carotene Smoothie

Serves: 2

Prep Time: 5 minutes

Ingredients

2 carrots

4 cups raw spinach

½ cup light Greek yogurt

½ tsp cinnamon

½ cup ice

Directions

- Steam spinach.
- Place all ingredients in NUTRiBULLET and mix until smooth.

Nutrition (g)

Calories 103

Fat 3

Sodium 136 (mg)

Carbs 14

Fiber 3

Sugars 8

Protein6

The Super Slim and Strong

Serves: 2

Prep Time: 5 minutes

Ingredients

4 cups fresh kale

2 tbsp chia seeds

2 tbsp sunflower seeds

½ cup pomegranate juice

½ cup ice

Directions

- o Steam your spinach prior to making your smoothie and allow it to cool.
- o Place all ingredients in NUTRiBULLET and mix until smooth.

Nutrition (g)

Calories 103

Fat 3

Sodium 136 (mg)

Carbs 14

Sugars 8

Protein 6

The Chocolate Orange Smoothie

Serves: 2

Prep Time: 5 minutes

Ingredients

1 large orange, peeled, segmented

1 banana

1 tbsp cocoa powder

½ cup almond milk

1/2 cup ice

Directions

- o Place ingredients in NUTRiBULLET and mix until smooth.

Nutrition (g)

Calories 240

Fat 15

Sodium 10 (mg)

Carbs 29

Sugars 18

Protein 3

The Green Weight Slam Smoothie

Serves: 2

Prep Time: 5 minutes

Ingredients

4 cups fresh spinach

4 cups fresh kale

3 kiwi fruit, skin removed

2 limes, juiced

1 tsp wheatgrass

½ cup ice

Directions

- o Steam both the kale and spinach and cool.
- o Place all ingredients in NUTRiBULLET and mix until smooth.

Nutrition (g)

Calories 169

Fat 1

Sodium 112 (mg)

Carbs 40

Sugars 12

Protein 7

The Cantaloupe Smoothie

Serves: 2

Prep Time: 5 minutes

Ingredients

1 cup cantaloupe

½ cup coconut water

¼ tsp red chili pepper flakes

1 tbsp honey

Directions

- ○ Place ingredients in NUTRiBULLET and mix until smooth.

Nutrition (g)

Calories 32

Fat 0

Sodium (0) g

Carbs 9

Sugars 9

Protein 0

Chapter 4: Healthy Heart Smoothies

Your heart works long hours every single day of the year and it's got a big job to do. The heart is responsible for making sure your whole body Is running like a well-oiled machine.

The heart's job is to pump blood to all areas of your body, and this is vital because that's how your organs get the nutrients they need to keep going. The blood also helps to clean the gunk out of your body by carrying it away from your organs

Clearly, the heart's doing an important job and the good news is that you can help by eating the right things. The food you put into your body is the equivalent of the oil you put into your car. If you put good food in, your body will run beautifully.

In order to help the heart do its thing, you're going to want to eat raspberries and blueberries for the amazing antioxidant components that help slam cell-damaging free radicals out of your body. When you're eating food full of antioxidants you're helping to ensure there is no build up of gunk in your system – which can clog up your arteries and make it difficult for the heart to pump.

You also want to incorporate good fats like avocado and walnuts which raise the good HDL cholesterol in your body and reduce the bad LDL.

Eating bananas and other sources of potassium like dairy is great for your heart because it can help to lower blood pressure.

Eating citrus is especially important for women when it comes to heart health as studies have concluded that it could reduce the chances of stroke. Additionally, citrus fruit are a great source of antioxidants which does your whole body good.

The following smoothies are all made up of ingredients that are going to help ensure your heart is pumping clean and pure all day long.

Grapefruit Smoothie

Serves: 2

Prep Time: 5 minutes

Ingredients

1 grapefruit

½ avocado, pitted

1 cucumber

½ cup of ice

Directions

- Separate grapefruit segments from peel.
- Place ingredients in NUTRiBULLET and mix until smooth.

Nutrition (g)

Calories 146

Fat 10

Sodium 8 (mg)

Carbs 15

Fiber 5

Sugars 7

Protein 2

Grapefruit Passion Smoothie

Serves: 2

Prep Time: 5 minutes

Ingredients

1 grapefruit

1 passionfruit

¼ cup mint leaves

½ cup orange juice

½ cup ice

Directions

- o Place ingredients in NUTRiBULLET and mix until smooth.

Nutrition (g)

Calories 54

Fat 0

Sodium 6(mg)

Carbs 13

Fiber 2

Sugars 10

Protein 1

Blueberry Passion Smoothie

Serves: 2

Prep Time: 5 minutes

Ingredients

1 cup blueberries

1 tsp wheatgrass

½ cup ice

¼ tsp vanilla

Directions

- ○ Place ingredients in NUTRiBULLET and mix until smooth.

Nutrition (g)

Calories 46

Fat 0

Sodium 2 (mg)

Carbs 11

Fiber 2

Sugars 8

Protein 1

Peach Walnut Smoothie

Serves: 2

Prep Time: 5 minutes

Ingredients

½ cup walnut, chopped

2 peaches, pitted, skin-removed

½ cup low-fat yogurt

½ cup ice

Directions

- o Place ingredients in NUTRiBULLET and mix until smooth.

Nutrition (g)

Calories 275

Fat 19

Sodium 45 (mg)

Carbs 17

Fiber 4

Sugars 13

Protein 12

Raspberry Almond Smoothie

Serves: 2

Prep Time: 5 minutes

Ingredients

½ cup raspberries

½ cup blanched almonds

½ cup low-fat Greek yogurt

½ cup ice

1 cardamom pod

Directions

- ○ Blanche almonds overnight, remove skin.
- ○ Remove cardamom seeds from pod, throw out pod.
- ○ Place ingredients in NUTRiBULLET and mix until smooth.

Nutrition (g)

Calories 214

Fat 13

Sodium 35 (mg)

Carbs 20

Fiber 5

Sugars 14

Protein 8

Citrus Avocado Smoothie

Serves: 2

Prep Time: 5 minutes

Ingredients

2 large oranges

½ avocado, pitted, skin-removed1 cucumber

3/4 cup of ice

Directions

- ○ Separate orange segments from peel.

- Place ingredients in NUTRiBULLET and mix until smooth.

Nutrition (g)

Calories 189

Fat 10

Sodium 6 (mg)

Carbs 26

Fiber 8

Sugars 17

Protein 3

Berry Trio Smoothie

Serves: 2

Prep Time: 5 minutes

Ingredients

½ cup frozen strawberries

½ cup frozen blueberries

½ cup frozen raspberries

½ cup ice

½ tsp vanilla

Directions

- Place ingredients in NUTRiBULLET and mix until smooth.

Nutrition (g)

Calories 104

Fat 2

Sodium 4 (mg)

Carbs 20

Fiber 4

Sugars 4

Protein 3

Strawberry Oatmeal Smoothie

Serves: 2

Prep Time: 5 minutes

Ingredients

½ cup oatmeal, prepared

1 cup strawberries, husked

½ cup ice

½ tsp vanilla

Directions

- o Place ingredients in NUTRiBULLET and mix until smooth.

Nutrition (g)

Calories 104

Fat 2

Sodium 4 (mg)

Carbs 20

Fiber 4

Sugars 4

Protein 3

Mint Chocolate Smoothie

Serves: 2

Prep Time: 5 minutes

Ingredients

¼ cup min leaves

1/3 cup bitter chocolate (70%)

½ cup low-fat vanilla yogurt

1/4 cup walnut, chopped

½ cup ice

Directions

- Place ingredients in NUTRiBULLET and mix until smooth.

Nutrition (g)

Calories 151

Fat 10

Sodium 45 (mg)

Carbs 6

Fiber 1

30

Sugars 5

Protein 7

Papaya Avocado Smoothie

Serves: 2

Prep Time: 5 minutes

Ingredients

½ cup papaya

½ cup avocado, pitted, skin-removed

½ cup low-fat Greek yogurt

½ cup ice

Directions

- o Place ingredients in NUTRiBULLET and mix until smooth.

Nutrition (g)

Calories 151

Fat 8

Sodium 39 (mg)

Carbs 19

Fiber 3

Sugars 14

Protein 3

Chapter 5: Detoxification & Cleansing Smoothies

You take a shower every single day, but how about that shower for the inside of your body – most people forget that it's important to. Over time, toxins can build up inside of your body and if left that way for too long, they can cause serious damage. It is important to eat foods that cleanse our body and even give your body a true cleansing twice a year with a detox program.

The following recipes have been concocted to help you keep your body clean every single day and if you want to do a detox you can drink any combination of the following recipes for 3 to 5 days to cleanse out your system and give your body a toxin free restart. You'll feel light, clean and kind of airy like you're a clean cloud just floating amongst humans.

The Detox Smoothie

Serves: 2

Prep Time: 5 minutes

Ingredients

1 cup cranberries, pitted

2 lemons, juiced

½ cup ice

3 leaves mint

Directions

- o Place ingredients in NUTRiBULLET and mix until smooth.

Nutrition (g)

Calories 47

Fat 0

Sodium 3 (mg)

Carbs 10

Fiber 4

Sugars4

Protein 0

The Blue Gods Smoothie

Serves: 2

Prep Time: 5 minutes

Ingredients

1 cup blueberries

2 lemons, juiced

1 tbsp ginger, grated

½ cup ice

Directions

- o Place ingredients in NUTRiBULLET and mix until smooth.

Nutrition (g)

Calories 68

Fat 0

Sodium 4 (mg)

Carbs 18

Fiber 4

Sugars 9

Protein 1

Citrus Chili Antioxidant Smoothie

Serves: 2

Prep Time: 5 minutes

Ingredients

1 orange

1 grapefruit

1 lemon

1 green chili pepper

½ cup ice

Directions

- o Place ingredients in NUTRiBULLET and mix until smooth.

Nutrition (g)

Calories 73

Fat 0

Sodium 3 (mg)

Carbs 19

Fiber 4

Sugars 14

Protein 2

Fiber Flush Smoothie

Serves: 2

Prep Time: 5 minutes

Ingredients

3/4 cup broccoli florets

1/3 cup blackberries

½ avocado

½ cup ice

1 tsp Stevia powder (if desired)

Directions

- Place ingredients in NUTRiBULLET and mix until smooth.

Nutrition (g)

Calories 124

Fat 10

Sodium 16 (mg)

Carbs 9

Fiber 6

Sugars 2

Protein 2

Pear Detox Smoothie

Serves: 2

Prep Time: 5 minutes

Ingredients

2 pears, stemmed, seeded

1 lemon, peel-removed

1/2 cup coconut water

¼ cup ice

Directions

- o Place ingredients in NUTRiBULLET and mix until smooth.

Nutrition (g)

Calories 159

Fat 0

Sodium 16 (mg)

Carbs 42

Fiber 7

Sugars 29

Protein 1

Cran-Apple Detox

Serves: 2

Prep Time: 5 minutes

Ingredients

2 green apples

½ cup organic cranberry juice

1 lemon, juiced

2 tsp organic honey

¾ cup iced

Directions

- o Place ingredients in NUTRiBULLET and mix until smooth.

Nutrition (g)

Calories 139

Fat 0

Sodium 5 (mg)

Carbs 36

Fiber 6

Sugars 26

Protein 1

Lime Barley Flush Smoothie

Serves: 2

Prep Time: 5 minutes

Ingredients

1/3 cup barley

1 pear

2 limes, juiced

½ cup coconut water

½ cup ice

Directions

- o Place ingredients in NUTRiBULLET and mix until smooth.

Nutrition (g)

Calories 184

Fat 1

Sodium 14 (mg)

Carbs 44

Fiber 9

Sugars 12

Protein 5

Blueberry Orange Smoothie

Serves: 2

Prep Time: 5 minutes

Ingredients

1 orange, peel-removed

1/3 cup blueberries

1/3 cup barley

1 tsp ground flaxseed

½ cup coconut water

½ cup ice

Directions

- o Place ingredients in NUTRiBULLET and mix until smooth.

Nutrition (g)

Calories 187

Fat 1

Sodium 12 (mg)

Carbs 41

Fiber 8

Sugars 15

Protein 5

Green Detox Smoothie

Serves: 2

Prep Time: 5 minutes

Ingredients

1/2 English cucumber

2 limes

1/3 cup mint

1/3

 cup coconut water

1/3 cup ice

1 tbsp honey

Directions

○ Place ingredients in NUTRiBULLET and mix until smooth.

Nutrition (g)

Calories 80

Fat 0

Sodium 13 (mg)

Carbs 22

Fiber 3

Sugars 14

Protein 2

Berry Detox Smoothie

Serves: 2

Prep Time: 5 minutes

Ingredients

½ cup blackberries

½ cup blueberries

1 lime, juiced

½ cup coconut water

½ cup ice

Directions

- o Place ingredients in NUTRiBULLET and mix until smooth.

Nutrition (g)

Calories 61

Fat 0

Sodium 9 (mg)

Carbs 16

Fiber 4

Sugars 10

Protein 1

Chapter 6: Energy Boost Smoothies

Food is energy, but the quality of energy varies from food to food, similar to the quality difference between discount batteries from the dollar store and batteries you're paying double digits for. One of those batteries is going to give you a burst of energy and then die out while the other will provide a steady stream of energy over a long period of time.

What you put into your body affects everything that you do and can be the reason behind a highly productive day versus a day you sleep walk though. The smoothies concocted for this section are especially designed to give you that extra energy boost when you're going hard and long all day.

The following smoothies have higher doses of fat and proteins than standard because these are the type of nutrients that take your body time to break down and in turn leave you feeling energized for longer.

Additionally, the following smoothies are made up of good heart-healthy fats which your body and brain need. Whip up one of the following smoothies for a pick-me-up or when you want to get powered-up until your next meal time.

The Banana Sprint Smoothie

Serves: 2

Prep Time: 5 minutes

Ingredients

1 banana

1/3 cup organic peanut butter

2 tbsp ground flaxseed

½ cup low-fat yogurt

¼ cup ice

Directions

- o Place ingredients in NUTRiBULLET and mix until smooth.

Nutrition (g)

Calories 386

Fat 25

Sodium 244 (mg)

Carbs 28

Fiber 6

Sugars16

Protein 16

The Spinach-Kale Super Energy Smoothie

Serves: 2

Prep Time: 15 minutes

Ingredients

4 cups fresh spinach

4 cups fresh kale

¼ cup pistachio nuts

1 egg

½ cup coconut milk

½ tsp vanilla

Directions

- o Steam spinach and kale, cool.
- o Place ingredients in NUTRiBULLET and mix until smooth.

Nutrition (g)

Calories 292

Fat 20

Sodium 185 (mg)

Carbs 22

Fiber 5

Sugars 3

Protein 11

The Chia Smoothie

Serves: 2

Prep Time: 5 minutes

Ingredients

2 tsp chia seeds

1/3 cup walnuts

4 Medjool dates, pitted

1 banana

3/4 cup low-fat yogurt

44

½ cup ice

Directions

○ Place ingredients in NUTRiBULLET and mix until smooth.

Nutrition (g)

Calories 256

Fat 14

Sodium 67 (mg)

Carbs 23

Fiber 4

Sugars 14

Protein 11

The Red Blast Smoothie

Serves: 2

Prep Time: 5 minutes

Ingredients

2 red beets, peeled

1 red apple

½ cup ice

1 tsp red chili pepper

Directions

- Place ingredients in NUTRiBULLET and mix until smooth.

Nutrition (g)

Calories 93

Fat 0

Sodium 80 (mg)

Carbs 23

Fiber 4

Sugars18

Protein 2

The Spiced Energy Smoothie

Serves: 2

Prep Time: 5 minutes

Ingredients

4 cups fresh kale

½ avocado, pitted, skin-removed

1 carrot

1 cup tomato juice

½ tsp salt

½ tsp black pepper

½ cup ice

Directions

- ○ Steam our kale.
- ○ Place ingredients in NUTRiBULLET and mix until smooth.

Nutrition (g)

Calories 203

Fat 10

Sodium 992 (mg)

Carbs 27

Fiber 7

Sugars 6

Protein 6

The Pomegranate Coconut

Smoothie

Serves: 2

Prep Time: 5 minutes

Ingredients

1 pomegranate

1 lemon, juiced

3/4 cup coconut milk

½ cup ice

Directions

- Place ingredients in NUTRiBULLET and mix until smooth.

Nutrition (g)

Calories 265

Fat 22

Sodium 16 (mg)

Carbs 21

Fiber 3

Sugars 14

Protein 3

Apple Nut Smoothie

Serves: 2

Prep Time: 5 minutes

Ingredients

2 red apples, cored, stemmed

½ cup almond butter

½ tsp cinnamon

½ tsp vanilla

½ cup coconut water

Directions

- Place ingredients in NUTRiBULLET and mix until smooth.

Nutrition (g)

Calories 511

Fat 36

Sodium 8 (mg)

Carbs 41

Fiber 7

Sugars 23

Protein 14

Banana Muffin Smoothie

Serves: 2

Prep Time: 5 minutes

Ingredients

1 banana

1/3 cup walnuts

4 Medjool dates, pitted

3/4 cup low-fat yogurt

½ cup ice

Directions

- o Place ingredients in NUTRiBULLET and mix until smooth.

Nutrition (g)

Calories 287

Fat 14

Sodium 67(mg)

Carbs 33

Fiber 4

Sugars 23

Protein 11

Pumpkin Spice Smoothie

Serves: 2

Prep Time: 5 minutes

Ingredients

1 cup pumpkin cubes

1/2 cup coconut milk

½ filtered water

½ tsp cinnamon

½ tsp nutmeg

Directions

- o Place ingredients in NUTRiBULLET and mix until smooth.

Nutrition (g)

Calories 184

Fat 15

Sodium 15 (mg)

Carbs 14

Fiber 5

Sugars 6

Protein 3

Strawberry Chocolate Smoothie

Serves: 2

Prep Time: 5 minutes

Ingredients

½ cup frozen strawberries

1 banana

2 tbsp pure cocoa powder

½ avocado, pitted, skin-removed

½ cup coconut milk

1 tbsp Stevia

Directions

- o Place ingredients in NUTRiBULLET and mix until smooth.

Nutrition (g)

Calories 321

Fat 25

Sodium 13 (mg)

Carbs 26

Fiber 8

Sugars 12

Protein 4

Chapter 7: Radiant Skin smoothies

There are few things that can make or break first impression like the health of your skin can. The first thing people will notice about you when they meet you is that one giant body part that covers all of you. If your skin is normal, they'll move on to evaluate other parts of you, but if it's dry and flaky that is what they will remember. Sporting terrible skin sends people a negative message, one that says you don't take care of yourself so how could you possibly take care of anything else.

First impressions matter!

The good news is that making some changes in your diet can make a massive difference in the way your skin looks and feels. So we've created a delicious bucket list of smoothies you're going to want to incorporate into your skin-aware lifestyle.

The following smoothies are great for your skin because they're chock full of things like antioxidants which clear out all the gunk in your body that ends up on your skin in the form of pimples and other protrusions. The ingredients selected for these smoothies also hydrate you and provide you with the kind of good fats that will help you achieve baby soft skin.

Drink one of these radiant smoothies daily and see a massive difference in just 10 days, you're going to be glowing all over the place.

The Watermelon Mint Smoothie

Serves: 2

Prep Time: 5 minutes

Ingredients

1-1/2 cup watermelon

¼ cup mint leaves

¼ cup ice

2 tsp agave nectar

Directions

- o Place ingredients in NUTRiBULLET and mix until smooth.

Nutrition (g)

Calories 88

Fat 0

Carbs 23

Sugars 20

Protein 1

The Shine On Blueberry Smoothie

Serves: 2

Prep Time: 5 minutes

Ingredients

1 cup blueberries

4 tbsp pomegranate nectar

2 lemons, juiced

½ cup ice

2 tsp agave nectar

Directions

- o Place ingredients in NUTRiBULLET and mix until smooth.

Nutrition (g)

Calories 117

Fat 1

Carbs 32

Sugars 17

Protein 2

The Rosy Cheeks Smoothie

Serves: 2

Prep Time: 5 minutes

Ingredients

1 pomegranate

1 lemon, juiced

½ cup coconut water

1/2 cup ice

2 tsp agave nectar

Directions

- o Place ingredients in NUTRiBULLET and mix until smooth.

Nutrition (g)

Calories 73

Fat 0

Carbs 19

Sugars 15

Protein 1

The Ginger Cleanse Smoothie

Serves: 2

Prep Time: 5 minutes

Ingredients

2" chunk ginger, peeled

2 oranges, segmented

2 tsp chia seeds

¾ cup ice

Directions

- o Place ingredients in NUTRiBULLET and mix until smooth.

Nutrition (g)

Calories 73

Fat 0

Carbs 19

Sugars 15

Protein 1

The Avocado Nourishment Smoothie

Serves: 2

Prep Time: 5 minutes

Ingredients

½ avocado, pitted, skin-removed

1 grapefruit, peeled, segmented

2 tbsp flaxseed, ground

½ cup coconut milk

½ cup ice

2 tsp agave nectar

Directions

- o Place ingredients in NUTRiBULLET and mix until smooth.

Nutrition (g)

Calories 278

Fat 26

Carbs 10

Sugars 2

Protein 4

The Beta Smoothie

Serves: 2

Prep Time: 5 minutes

Ingredients

3 carrots, peeled

1/2 cup walnuts

½ cup coconut milk

½ tsp cardamom

2 tsp agave nectar

Directions

- o Place ingredients in NUTRiBULLET and mix until smooth.

Nutrition (g)

Calories 370

Fat 33

Carbs 16

Sugars 7

Protein 10

The Orange Green Tea Smoothie

Serves: 2

Prep Time: 5 minutes

Ingredients

1 large orange, segmented

3/4 cup brewed green tea

½ cup soy milk

½ tsp vanilla bean

¼ cup ice

1 tsp Stevia

Directions

- o Cool tea.
- o Place all ingredients into NUTRiBULLET and mix until smooth.

Nutrition (g)

Calories 123

Fat 1

Carbs 27

Sugars 19

Protein 4

The Rose Hip Smoothie

Serves: 2

Prep Time: 5 minutes

Ingredients

1 cup Rose Hip Tea

1 lemon juiced

2 scoops Vanilla protein powder

1 cup ice

2 tsp agave nectar

Directions

- Place ingredients in NUTRiBULLET and mix until smooth.

Nutrition (g)

Calories 188

Fat 2

Carbs 23

Sugars 17

Protein 23

The Balsamic Cleanse Smoothie

Serves: 2

Prep Time: 5 minutes

Ingredients

3 tbsp balsamic vinegar

2 medium tomatoes, stemmed

2 tbsp flaxseed ground

2 limes, juiced

½ cup ice

½ tsp sea salt

½ tsp black pepper

Directions

- Place ingredients in NUTRiBULLET and mix until smooth.

Nutrition (g)

Calories 88

Fat 3

Carbs 15

Sugars 4

Protein 3

The Coconut Smoothie

Serves: 2

Prep Time: 5 minutes

Ingredients

1 peach, pitted

1/2 cup walnuts

1 cup coconut milk

½ tsp vanilla bean

Directions

- o Place ingredients in NUTRiBULLET and mix until smooth.

Nutrition (g)

Calories 488

Fat 47

Carbs 14

Sugars 9

Protein 11

Those of you living with diabetes are required to be extra vigilant when it comes to what you consume and that can be hard work. Some folks are so vigilant about their intake that they've deemed smoothies as no-no's due to possibly high sugar content. In some cases it is true that the sugar content of smoothies can be high, particularly when you're purchasing from a restaurant or fast food joint. However, when you make those smoothies at home, you can control everything and that includes the sugar content.

In fact, all you really need to do is avoid adding any extra sugar in addition to your whole foods smoothie content and you should be just fine. We'll be using a mix of fruits and veggies in the following recipes which means you will be consuming natural sugars. Although natural sugars are much better for you than synthetic ones, you should calculate the consumption of these sugars into your daily sugar/carb count.

If you feel a particular smoothie has a little bit more fruit than you can handle, just reduce the fruit and a little more of the liquid ingredient. If the recipe calls for veggies and fruits, you can up the veg and lower the fruit depending on your particular needs.

The Green Force Smoothie

Serves: 2

Prep Time: 5 minutes

Ingredients

8 cups spinach

Handful fresh basil leaves

2 limes, juiced

3 tsp rapeseed oil

3/4 cup ice

Directions

- o Steam spinach and cool.
- o Place ingredients in NUTRiBULLET and mix until smooth.

Nutrition (g)

Calories 116

Fat 8

Carbs 12

Sugars 2

Protein 4

The Pear Nut Smoothie

Serves: 2

Prep Time: 5 minutes

Ingredients

2 pears, cored

1 cup soy milk

¼ cup ice

Directions

- o Place ingredients in NUTRiBULLET and mix until smooth.

Nutrition (g)

Calories 170

Fat 2

Carbs 38

Sugars 24

Protein 4

The Sour Apple Smoothie

Serves: 2

Prep Time: 5 minutes

Ingredients

2 green apples, cored

3 lemons, juiced

½ cup coconut water

½ cup ice

Directions

- o Place ingredients in NUTRiBULLET and mix until smooth.

Nutrition (g)

Calories 112

Fat 0

Carbs 28

Sugars 22

Protein 1

Pink Grapefruit Smoothie

Serves: 2

Prep Time: 5 minutes

Ingredients

1 pink grapefruit, peeled, segmented

¼ cup raspberries

1/2 cup coconut water

½ cup ice

Directions

- o Place ingredients in NUTRiBULLET and mix until smooth.

Nutrition (g)

Calories 43

Fat 0

Carbs 11

Sugars 9

Protein 1

The Banana Raisin Smoothie

Serves: 2

Prep Time: 5 minutes

Ingredients

1 banana

¼ cup raisins

¼ cup almonds

¾ cup coconut milk

½ tsp vanilla beans

Directions

- o Place ingredients in NUTRiBULLET and mix until smooth.

Nutrition (g)

Calories 228

Fat 8

Carbs 36

Sugars 22

Protein 7

The Peanut Smoothie

Serves: 2

Prep Time: 5 minutes

Ingredients

2 tbsp unsalted peanut butter

25g bittersweet chocolate

¾ cup low-fat milk

½ tsp vanilla bean

Directions

- Place ingredients in NUTRiBULLET and mix until smooth.

Nutrition (g)

Calories 208

Fat 12

Carbs 15

Sugars 12

Protein 9

The Citrus Smoothie

Serves: 2

Prep Time: 5 minutes

Ingredients

2 oranges, peeled, segmented

1 lime, juiced

1 lemon, juiced

½ cup coconut water

½ cup ice

Directions

- Place ingredients in NUTRiBULLET and mix until smooth.

68

Nutrition (g)

Calories 116

Fat 0

Carbs 30

Sugars 20

Protein 3

The Pumpkin Spice Smoothie

Serves: 2

Prep Time: 5 minutes

Ingredients

1 cup steamed pumpkin

½ cup coconut milk

½ cup ice

½ tsp cinnamon

½ tsp nutmeg

Directions

- o Place ingredients in NUTRiBULLET and mix until smooth.

Nutrition (g)

Calories 184

Fat 15

Carbs 14

Sugars 6

Protein 3

The Coffee Date Smoothie

Serves: 2

Prep Time: 5 minutes

Ingredients

1 cup good-quality brewed coffee

4 Medjool dates, pitted

½ cup coconut milk

½ cup ice

Directions

- o Place ingredients in NUTRiBULLET and mix until smooth.

Nutrition (g)

Calories 219

Fat 14

Carbs 24

Sugars 20

Protein 3

The Kale Strong Smoothie

Serves: 2

Prep Time: 5 minutes

Ingredients

4 cups fresh kale

2 tsp wheatgrass

½ cup lettuce

1 banana

½ tsp vanilla bean

½ cup ice

Directions

- o Steam kale, set aside to cool.
- o Once kale is cool, place all ingredients in NUTRiBULLET and mix until smooth.

Nutrition (g)

Calories 128

Fat 0

Carbs 29

Sugars 8

Protein 6

Chapter 9: Low Carb Superfood Smoothies

It's no secret that when you drop the carbs, you drop that excess weight. Simple carbohydrates are used up by our bodies easily and quickly because they're simple to breakdown. This also means that your blood sugar levels spike when you eat simple carbs.

On the other hand it takes your body a lot more work to break down proteins, and in particular, fats to use as energy. When you significantly eliminate carbs, your body goes into ketosis, which means it starts using fats for energy instead of carbohydrates.

Once it starts using fats for energy, it also begins to use those stored up fats and in turn you start shedding weight fast.

Beyond the weight control aspect, low carb foods make you feel fuller longer and in turn provide you with much more energy for longer periods of time.

The following smoothies have been designed in true low-carb fashion with reduced sugars and replacement of dairy products with nut and soy milks. You are guaranteed to get a sweet and lasting energy boost from this section of smoothies.

The Kale Mango Smoothie

Serves: 2

Prep Time: 5 minutes

Ingredients

1 cup diced mango

6 cups fresh kale

½ cup mint leaves

1 cup coconut water

Directions

- o   Steam kale and cool.
- o   Remove pit and peel from mango.
- o   Place ingredients in NUTRiBULLET and mix until smooth.

Nutrition (g)

Calories 153

Fat 1

Carbs 35

Sugars 22

Protein 4

The Mango Smoothie

Serves: 2

Prep Time: 5 minutes

Ingredients

1 mango

2 cups fresh kale

½ cup mint leaves

1 cup coconut water

Directions

- Place ingredients in NUTRiBULLET and mix until smooth.

Nutrition (g)

Calories 131

Fat 0

Carbs 30

Sugars 19

Protein

The Papaya Green Smoothie

Serves: 2

Prep Time: 5 minutes

Ingredients

1 papaya

1 lemon, juiced6

6 cups fresh spinach

1 cup coconut water

Directions

- Steam spinach and cool.
- Remove skin from papaya, pit and roughly cut them up.
- ace ingredients in NUTRiBULLET and mix until smooth.

Nutrition (g)

Calories 119

Fat 1

Carbs 28

Sugars 16

Protein 5

Celery Refresher Smoothie

Serves: 2

Prep Time: 5 minutes

Ingredients

3 celery stalks

2 tomatoes

2 tbsp chia seeds

¼ cup cilantro leaves

½ tsp salt

½ tsp black pepper

½ cup ice

Directions

- o Place ingredients in NUTRiBULLET and mix until smooth.

Nutrition (g)

Calories 184

Fat 10

Carbs 16

Sugars 4

Protein 8

The Strawberry Almond Smoothie

Serves: 2

Prep Time: 5 minutes

Ingredients

¾ cup strawberries, hulled

¾ cup Greek yogurt

½ cup ice

½ tsp vanilla beans

Directions

- o Place ingredients in NUTRiBULLET and mix until smooth.

Nutrition (g)

Calories 96

Fat 2

Carbs 8

Sugars 7

Protein 10

The Choco-Nut Smoothie

Serves: 2

Prep Time: 5 minutes

Ingredients

1/2 cup almonds

2 tbsp flaxseed

3 tbsp cacao powder

½ cup almond milk

¾ cup ice

1 tsp Stevia

Directions

- o Place ingredients in NUTRiBULLET and mix until smooth.

Nutrition (g)

Calories 331

Fat 30

Carbs 15

Sugars 3

Protein 9

The Pistachio Raspberry Smoothie

Serves: 2

Prep Time: 5 minutes

Ingredients

1 cup pistachio nuts in the shell

1/2 cup frozen raspberries

¾ cup coconut milk

½ tsp cardamom

Directions

- o Place ingredients in NUTRiBULLET and mix until smooth.

Nutrition (g)

Calories 313

Fat 29

Carbs 13

Sugars 5

Protein 6

The Thai Cucumber Smoothie

Serves: 2

Prep Time: 5 minutes

Ingredients

1 cucumber

2 limes, juiced

3/4 cup coconut milk

¼ cup ice

1 tsp Stevia

Directions

- o Place ingredients in NUTRiBULLET and mix until smooth.

Nutrition (g)

Calories

Fat

Carbs

Sugars

Protein

Apple Date Smoothie

Serves: 2

Prep Time: 5 minutes

Ingredients

1 red apple, cored, stemmed

2 tbsp flax seeds

7 oz Greek yogurt

½ cup ice

½ tsp cinnamon

Directions

- o Place ingredients in NUTRiBULLET and mix until smooth.

Nutrition (g)

Calories 161

Fat 4

Carbs 19

Sugars 14

Protein 12

The Tangerine Creamsicle Smoothie

Serves: 2

Prep Time: 5 minutes

Ingredients

2 Tangerines, peeled

1 cup coconut milk

½ tsp vanilla bean

¼ cup ice

Directions

- o Place ingredients in NUTRiBULLET and mix until smooth.

Nutrition (g)

Calories 324

Fat 29

Carbs 18

Sugars 13

Protein 3

Chapter 10: Antioxidant Smoothies

Antioxidants are superheroes in the body world. Antioxidants help to prevent the spread of free radicals and it is those radicals that can wreak havoc in your body, causing you to physically age faster as well as look a whole lot older too.

Free radicals attach themselves to healthy molecule causing a ripple reaction that ends up destroying cells and creating a whole lot more free radicals. Antioxidants pounce on these radical bullies and get rid of them. Ensuring you have enough antioxidants in your diet is important since not only will you look better, but you'll feel better too.

The smoothies in the following chapter are chock full of antioxidants like those found in oranges, grapefruits, berries and more. Our antioxidant smoothies will help you glow from the inside out.

Pomegranate Panache Smoothie

Serves: 2

Prep Time: 5 minutes

Ingredients

1 pomegranate

1 lemon, juiced

½ cup ice

½ cup coconut water

Directions

- Separate pomegranate arils from rind and place arils in NUTRiBULLET.

- Add remaining ingredients and mix until well combined.

Nutrition (g)

Calories 70

Fat 0

Carbs18

Sugars 13

Protein 1

The Lemon Drop Smoothie

Serves: 2

Prep Time: 5 minutes

Ingredients

2 lemons

½ cup mint leaves

¾ cup coconut milk

½ cup ice

1 tsp Stevia

Directions

- Place ingredients in NUTRiBULLET and mix until smooth.

Nutrition (g)

Calories 230

Fat 22

Carbs 8

Sugars 3

Protein 3

The Green Antioxidant Smoothie

Serves: 2

Prep Time: 5 minutes

Ingredients

6 cups fresh spinach

¼ cup parsley

1 orange

½ cup ice

½ cup coconut water

Directions

- o Steam spinach and cool.
- o Place ingredients in NUTRiBULLET and mix until smooth.

Nutrition (g)

Calories 77

Fat 1

Carbs 17

Sugars 12

Protein 4

The Blueberry Shake Smoothie

Serves: 2

Prep Time: 5 minutes

Ingredients

1 cup frozen blue berries

2 scoops vanilla protein powder

½ cup coconut milk

½ cup ice

1 tsp Stevia

Directions

- o Place ingredients in NUTRiBULLET and mix until smooth.

Nutrition (g)

Calories 299

Fat 16

Carbs 19

Sugars 10

Protein 24

The Raspberry Chocolate Smoothie

Serves: 2

Prep Time: 5 minutes

Ingredients

½ cup raspberries

3 tbsp cacao powder

¾ cup soy milk

½ cup ice

Directions

- o Place ingredients in NUTRiBULLET and mix until smooth.

Nutrition (g)

Calories 87

Fat 3

Carbs 13

Sugars 5

Protein 5

Grapefruit Smoothie

Serves: 2

Prep Time: 5 minutes

Ingredients

1 pink grapefruit, segmented

½ cup cilantro leaves

½ cup coconut water

½ cup ice

2 tbsp honey

Directions

- o Place ingredients into NUTRiBULLET and blend.

Nutrition (g)

Calories 96

Fat 0

Carbs 25

Sugars 24

Protein 1

The Carrot Spice Smoothie

Serves: 2

Prep Time: 5 minutes

Ingredients

3 carrots, peeled

1 cup coconut milk

½ cup ice

1/3 tsp cinnamon powder

1/3 tsp nutmeg

1 tsp Stevia

Directions

- o Place ingredients in NUTRiBULLET and mix until smooth.

Nutrition (g)

Calories 317

Fat 29

Carbs 17

Sugars 9

Protein 4

The Spiced Lemonade Smoothie

Serves: 2

Prep Time: 5 minutes

Ingredients

3 lemons

1 tsp hot chili powder

½ tsp turmeric½ cup ice

1/2 cup freshly squeezed orange juice

½ cup coconut water

½ cup ice

2 tbsp organic honey

Directions

- o Place ingredients in NUTRiBULLET and mix until smooth.

Nutrition (g)

Calories 217

Fat 1

Carbs 55

Sugars 51

Protein 1

The Avocado Orange Smoothie

Serves: 2

Prep Time: 5 minutes

Ingredients

½ avocado, pitted, peeled

1 orange, peeled

1/2 cup yogurt

½ tsp vanilla bean

Directions

- o Place ingredients in NUTRiBULLET and mix until smooth.

Nutrition (g)

Calories 192

Fat 11

Carbs 21

Sugars 13

Protein 5

The Kiwi Berry Smoothie

Serves: 2

Prep Time: 5 minutes

Ingredients

3 kiwi fruit, peeled

½ cup frozen blueberries

1 tbsp wheatgrass

½ cup brewed green tea

2 tbsp honey

Directions

- ○ Place ingredients in NUTRiBULLET and mix until smooth.

Nutrition (g)

Calories 157

Fat 1

Carbs 40

Sugars 31

Protein 2

Chapter 11: Anti-aging Smoothies

What you put into your body is who you are. The ingredients that make you are also the ingredients that can break you and that is why it is so very important that you eat according to how you want to live. If you want to live a young, healthy life, you must eat foods that promote vitality and rejuvenation. Conversely, if you don't mind aging fast and slowing down, then you can go ahead and eat boxed, sugary, oily foods lacking in everything but taste.

Now, if you're on the young and healthy team (and we believe you are), then these anti-aging smoothies we've created are for you. The ingredients have been selected for particular qualities that promote anti-aging of your body and mind. We've given each one a name that denotes what that smoothie will target, however all of the smoothies in this section will assist in reducing cell damage that ultimately leads to aging.

These NUTRiBULLET smoothies are set to stop that clock of yours and even do a little rewind.

Eye Health Smoothie

Serves: 2

Prep Time: 5 minutes

Ingredients

4 carrots, stemmed

4 ml gingko biloba extract

2 tbsp honey

½ tsp cinnamon

½ tsp nutmeg

½ cup ice

½ cup coconut milk

Directions

- o Place ingredients in NUTRiBULLET and mix until smooth.

Nutrition (g)

Calories 256

Fat 15

Carbs 33

Sugars 25

Protein 3

Collagen Protection Smoothie

Serves: 2

Prep Time: 5 minutes

Ingredients

2 medium tomatoes, stemmed

2 oranges, peeled

2 tbsp dry rosemary

¾ cup ice

Directions

- o Place ingredients in NUTRiBULLET and mix until smooth.

Nutrition (g)

Calories 120

Fat 1

Carbs 29

Sugars 20

Protein 3

Free Radical Fighting Smoothie

Serves: 2

Prep Time: 5 minutes

Ingredients

1-1/4 cup fresh blueberries

1 lemon, juiced

1 tbsp dried oregano or handful fresh

3/4 cup ice

Directions

- o Place ingredients in NUTRiBULLET and mix until smooth.

Nutrition (g)

Calories 67

Fat 1

Carbs 17

Sugars 10

Protein 1

Brain Boost Smoothie

Serves: 2

Prep Time: 5 minutes

Ingredients

1 cup mixed berries

2 tbsp flaxseed powder

2 scoops vanilla protein powder

2 tbsp honey

3/4 cup ice

Directions

- o Place ingredients in NUTRiBULLET and mix until smooth.

Nutrition (g)

Calories 294

Fat 6

Carbs 39

Sugars 24

Protein 25

Luscious Hair Smoothie

Serves: 2

Prep Time: 5 minutes

Ingredients

½ cup fresh mint leaves

3 tbsp cacao powder

1 avocado, pitted, peeled

2 tbsp honey

½ cup ice

Directions

- o Place ingredients in NUTRiBULLET and mix until smooth.

Nutrition (g)

Calories 298

Fat 21

Carbs 32

Sugars 18

Protein 4

Supple Skin Smoothie

Serves: 2

Prep Time: 5 minutes

Ingredients

1 tsp freshly-ground cinnamon

1 grapefruit

2 tbsp honey

½ cup coconut water

½ cup ice

Directions

- ○ Place ingredients into NUTRiBULLET and blend.

Nutrition (g)

Calories 98

Fat 0

Carbs 26

Sugars 25

Protein 1

Wrinkle-Away Smoothie

Serves: 2

Prep Time: 5 minutes

Ingredients

2 tbsp wheat germ

¼ cup Brazil Nuts

1/2 avocado, pitted, peeled

2 tbsp honey

½ cup Greek yogurt

½ cup coconut water

Directions

- ○ Place ingredients in NUTRiBULLET and mix until smooth.

Nutrition (g)

Calories 339

Fat 21

Carbs 32

Sugars 23

Protein 11

Nutrient Boost Smoothie

Serves: 2

Prep Time: 5 minutes

Ingredients

4 cups fresh kale

2 lemons, juiced

½ cup blueberries

½ tsp turmeric

4 ml. ginkgo biloba extract

½ cup coconut milk

½ cup ice

Directions

- o Steam kale.
- o Place ingredients in NUTRiBULLET and mix until smooth.

Nutrition (g)

Calories 244

Fat 15

Carbs 28

Sugars 7

Protein 6

Heart Health Smoothie

Serves: 2

Prep Time: 5 minutes

Ingredients

½ avocado, pitted, peeled

2 tbsp cacao powder

2 oranges, peeled

1 banana

½ cup ice

Directions

- o Place ingredients in NUTRiBULLET and mix until smooth.

Nutrition (g)

Calories 254

Fat 11

Carbs 42

Sugars 25

Protein 4

Bones So-Strong Smoothie

Serves: 2

Prep Time: 5 minutes

Ingredients

4 cups fresh spinach

2 egg yolks

2 tbsp honey

¾ cup vanilla Greek yogurt

¼ cup fresh orange juice

½ cup ice

Directions

- o Steam spinach.
- o Place all ingredients in NUTRiBULLET and mix until smooth.

Nutrition (g)

Calories 231

Fat 6

Carbs 34

Sugars 29

Protein 12

BONUS CHAPTER: Delicious NUTRiBULLET Soups

It is hard to believe that you can whip up a nutritious, delicious meal in a few minutes flat, but you absolutely can thanks to your shiny, new NUTRiBULLET.

Soups provide a great way to get wholesome veggies in your diet, but often times it means spending a lot of time hanging around a stove. However, with the NUTRiBULLET's super amped-up power we can create some great soups in under 5 minutes.

You are welcome to heat the soups up after you've whipped them into shape in your bullet or you can enjoy them cold. The wonderful thing here is that you can enjoy a quick savoury dish quickly, all you've got to do is add veggies and mix.

All of the soups we've created here are made up of simple and healthy ingredients – although we did get a little naughty with the Broccoli and Cheese Soup.

Enjoy these quick and delicious soups and we're sure you're going to be inspired to create some of your own.

Just veggie and go!

Sweet and Spicy Carrot Soup

Serves: 2

Prep Time: 5 minutes

Ingredients

4 carrots

2 cloves garlic

½ tsp red chili pepper

¼ tsp oregano

¼ tsp black pepper

¼ tsp salt

½ cup coconut milk

Directions

- o Combine ingredients in NUTRiBULLET, mix until smooth.

- o You can heat the soup up on your stovetop or enjoy cold in the summer.

Nutrition (g)

Calories 194

Fat 14

Carbs 17

Sugars 8

Protein 3

Gazpacho

Serves: 2

Prep Time: 5 minutes

Ingredients

2 medium tomatoes, stemmed

1/2 red bell pepper, seeded

½ small cucumber

½ small red onion, peeled

1 clove garlic, peeled

1 lemon, juiced

2 leaves fresh basil

1 tbsp extra virgin olive oil

¼ tsp cumin

¼ tsp black pepper

½ tsp salt

Directions

- o Place ingredients in NUTRiBULLET and give it a quick mix so you still have some texture in your super quick Gazpacho.

Nutrition (g)

Calories 122

Fat 8

Carbs 14

Sugars 7

Protein 3

Beet Soup

Serves: 2

Prep Time: 5 minutes

Ingredients

2 beets, quartered

1 lemon, juiced

½ tsp black pepper

1/2 cup low-sodium chicken stock

Salt to taste

Directions

- o Steam spinach and cool.
- o Place ingredients in NUTRiBULLET and mix until smooth.

Nutrition (g)

Calories 55

Fat 0

Carbs 13

Sugars 9

Protein 2

Red Lentil Soup

Serves: 2

Prep Time: 5 minutes

Ingredients

½ cup dry red lentils

1 small carrot

¼ tsp cumin

¼ tsp oregano

102

3/4 cup low-sodium chicken stock

Directions

- o   Soak lentils in hot water overnight.
- o   Place ingredients in NUTRiBULLET and mix until smooth.
- o   You can heat the soup up if desired or enjoy cold.

Nutrition (g)

Calories 183

Fat 0

Carbs 32

Sugars 2

Protein 13

Broccoli and Cheese Soup

Serves: 2

Prep Time: 5 minutes

Ingredients

1-1/4 cup broccoli florets

1/3 cup old cheddar cheese

½ cup low-sodium chicken stock

Salt to taste

Directions

- o   Place ingredients in NUTRiBULLET and mix until smooth.

○ Heat in pan over stovetop for a creamy soup.

Nutrition (g)

Calories 177

Fat 14

Carbs 3

Sugars 1

Protein 11

Conclusion:

If you've read through the whole book and tried each and every NUTRiBULLET smoothie, you my friend are probably are the healthiest person within a 100-mile radius. That also means you don't just wake up in the morning, you cartwheel out of bed, ready to hit the ground running thanks to all the energy you're getting from your smoothies.

Even if you haven't had a chance to try each and every smoothie, but are working them into your lifestyle, you will see a difference in your energy levels. Your energy increase is thanks to the fact that you're detoxifying your body and replacing some of the gunk that you were used to consuming with foods that are alive and in turn give you life energy.

The selection of NUTRiBULLET smoothies provided in this book will also help you drop pounds while giving you the fat you need to enjoy that supple skin we all want. And yes, smoothies aren't just great for looking good, they're also great in preventing numerous health conditions like diabetes. Once you start nourishing your body with the right foods, your body starts to work for you, not against you.

If you give your internal system all of the nutrients it needs to function well, you will see a difference in your overall health and your overall life. Using the NUTRiBULLET for your smoothie concoctions provides you with the extra benefit of the machine's extreme extracting abilities.

With NUTRiBULLET smoothies, you aren't just getting the nutrients from the flesh of your fruit or vegetable, but rather from the whole. And truth be told, the amount of fruits and veggies you'll get inside you with a smoothie is a lot more than you would by single servings.

The most important thing here is your health, after all you've only got one of you. So work these wonderful NUTRiBULLET smoothies into your daily nourishment schedule and watch your body thank you in all kinds of ways.

Here's to you, a glowing face and a happy life!

Now go Bullet!

I've had a personally enriching experience writing this book and hope that it translates to you too. Remember that I am with you at every step of this journey and have your back at all times. Finally, if you liked this book, then make sure you read my other books too. I guarantee that you'll be equally pleased with the experience.

The Paleo Diet

The Paleo diet, similar to the anti-inflammation diet works at eliminating foods that are difficult to digest (grains, legumes and dairy) and including foods that increase the consumption of vitamins, minerals and antioxidants. Known to improve blood lipids, promote weight loss and reduce pain from intestinal problems, the diet delivers on its promise of promoting good health and reducing intestinal problems. Intrigued and keen to more? You can purchase my book by visiting: coming soon

Anti Inflammatory Diet

Have you been experiencing diarrhea, abdominal cramps, mood swings, headaches, body pains, or insomnia?

Are you suffering from chronic inflammation and are keen to know more about the disease? Are you looking for anti-inflammatory foods and anti-inflammatory diet plans that deliver on their promise to cut back symptoms and give you some

respite? Finally, do you seek more control on the things that are currently affecting and impacting your life?

Well, if the answer is a resounding "YES", then you'll be happy to know that the key to understanding and overcoming your symptoms is just a click away.

Intrigued and want to know more?

If "YES" again, then your thirst for knowledge and answers has just been answered! This book has been specifically written for YOU!

You can purchase my book by visiting: http://www.amazon.com/dp/B01DPA99F8?ref_=pe_2427780_160035660

Bonus FREE Report – A gift from me to you

"6 Proven Health Benefits of Apple Cider Vinegar"

A miracle ingredient whose benefits range from healing skin allergies, killing harmful gut-bacteria, aiding digestion, controlling diabetes, reducing bad cholesterol, promoting weight loss, treating dandruff to preventing cancer and heart ailments, Apple Cider Vinegar is a versatile food component that goes beyond being just a cupboard-ingredient. In my book, I share with you the nutritional facts and beneficial properties of this highly handy fermented liquid. You can download my report by visiting: www.Freevinegar.com

Well, what are you waiting for? Make sure you grab a copy now!

Good luck!

Caroline

If you enjoyed this book can I please ask a favour, could you please leave me a review I would love to hear your feedback. It will only take a minute.

I thank you in advance

Made in the USA
Middletown, DE
18 June 2021